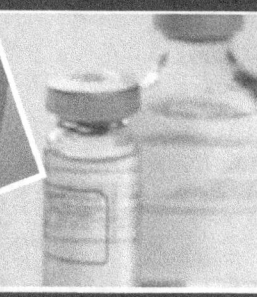

Kidney Failure

EAT RIGHT TO FEEL RIGHT

on Hemodialysis

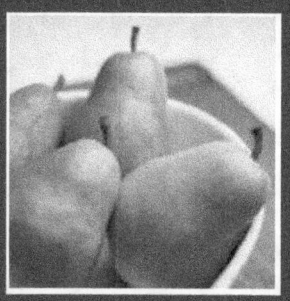

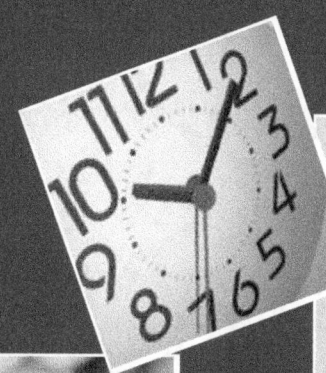

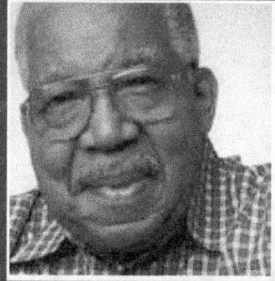

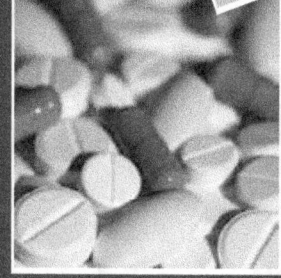

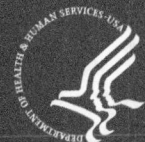

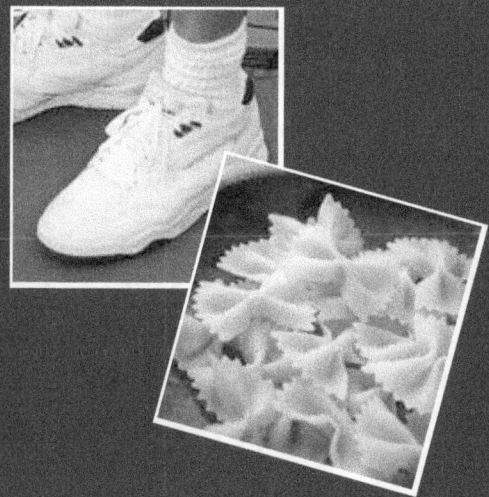

U.S. Department
of Health and
Human Services

NATIONAL INSTITUTES OF HEALTH

NIDDK | NATIONAL INSTITUTE OF
DIABETES AND DIGESTIVE
AND KIDNEY DISEASES

National Kidney and Urologic Diseases
Information Clearinghouse

Kidney Failure

EAT RIGHT TO FEEL RIGHT

on Hemodialysis

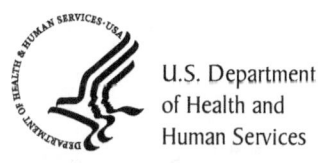

U.S. Department
of Health and
Human Services

NATIONAL INSTITUTES OF HEALTH

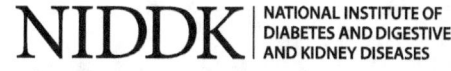

NATIONAL INSTITUTE OF
DIABETES AND DIGESTIVE
AND KIDNEY DISEASES

National Kidney and Urologic Diseases Information Clearinghouse

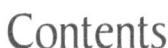

Contents

How to Use This Publication

When you start hemodialysis, you must make many changes in your life. Watching the foods you eat will make you healthier. This publication will help you choose the right foods.

Print this publication and use it with a dietitian to help you learn how to eat right to feel right on hemodialysis. Read one section at a time. Then go through the exercise for that section with your dietitian.

Once you have completed every exercise, keep a copy of this publication to remind yourself of foods you can eat and foods you need to avoid.

My dietitian's name is

_____

Phone

_____

How does food affect my hemodialysis?

Food gives you energy and helps your body repair itself. Food is broken down in your stomach and intestines. Your blood picks up nutrients from the digested food and carries them to all your body cells. These cells take nutrients from your blood and put waste products back into the bloodstream. When your kidneys were healthy, they worked around the clock to remove wastes from your blood. The wastes left your body when you urinated. Other wastes are removed in bowel movements.

Now that your kidneys have stopped working, hemodialysis removes wastes from your blood. But between dialysis sessions, wastes can build up in your blood and make you sick. You can reduce the amount of wastes by watching

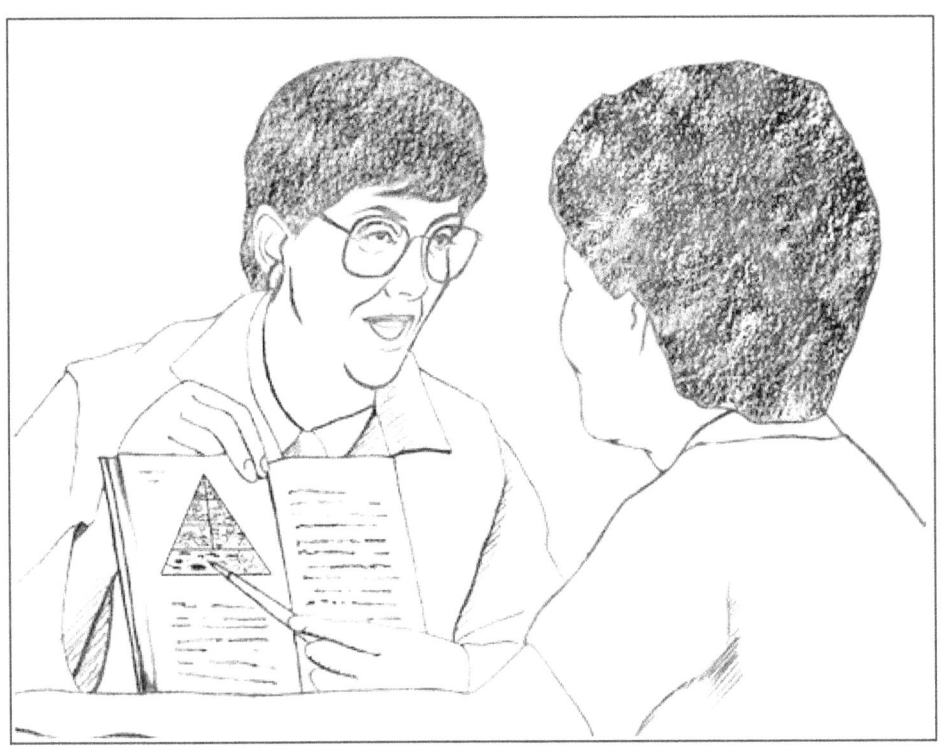

Talk with a dietitian to learn how to eat right on hemodialysis.

what you eat and drink. A good meal plan can improve your dialysis and your health.

Your clinic has a dietitian to help you plan meals. A dietitian specializes in food and nutrition. A dietitian with special training in care for kidney health is called a renal dietitian.

What do I need to know about fluids?

You already know you need to watch how much you drink. Any food that is liquid at room temperature also contains water. These foods include soup, Jell-O, and ice cream. Many fruits and vegetables contain lots of water, too. They include melons, grapes, apples, oranges, tomatoes, lettuce, and celery. All these foods add to your fluid intake.

Fluid can build up between dialysis sessions, causing swelling and weight gain. The extra fluid affects your blood pressure and can make your heart work harder. You could have serious heart trouble from overloading your system with fluid.

Control Your Thirst

The best way to reduce fluid intake is to reduce thirst caused by the salt you eat. Avoid salty foods like chips and pretzels. Choose low-sodium products.

You can keep your fluids down by drinking from smaller cups or glasses. Freeze juice in an ice cube tray and eat it like a popsicle. (Remember to count the popsicle in your fluid allowance!) The dietitian will be able to give you other tips for managing your thirst.

Your dry weight is your weight after a dialysis session when all of the extra fluid in your body has been removed. If you let too much fluid build up between sessions, it is harder to get down to your proper dry weight. Your dry weight may change over a period of 3 to 6 weeks. Talk with your doctor regularly about what your dry weight should be.

My dry weight should be _____.

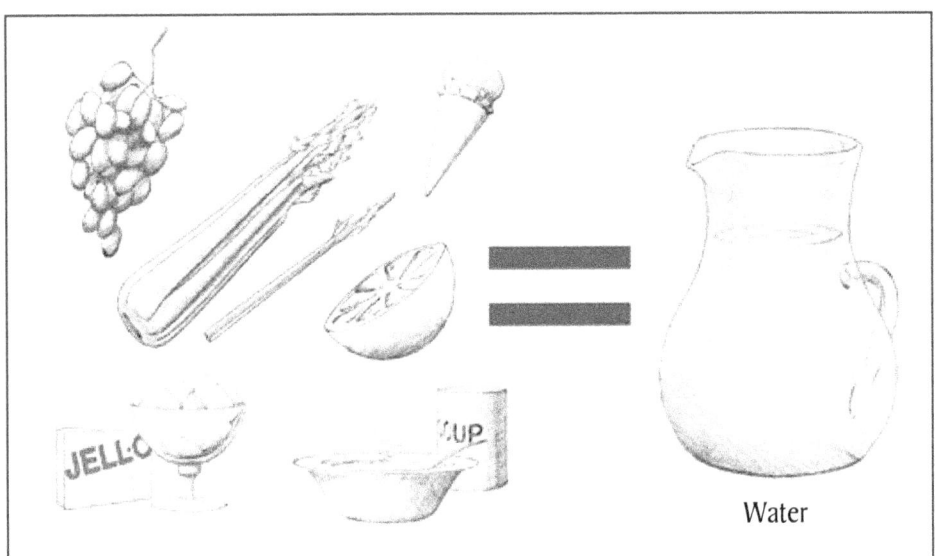

Many foods contain water.

Talk With a Dietitian

Even though you are on hemodialysis, your kidneys may still be able to remove some fluid. Or your kidneys may not remove any fluid at all. That is why every patient has a different daily allowance for fluid. Talk with your dietitian about how much fluid you can have each day.

I can have _____ ounces of fluid each day.

Plan 1 day of fluid servings:

I can have _____ ounce(s) of _____
with breakfast.

I can have _____ ounce(s) of _____
in the morning.

I can have _____ ounce(s) of _____
with lunch.

I can have _____ ounce(s) of _____
in the afternoon.

I can have _____ ounce(s) of _____
with supper.

I can have _____ ounce(s) of _____
in the evening.

TOTAL _____ ounces (should equal the allowance
written above)

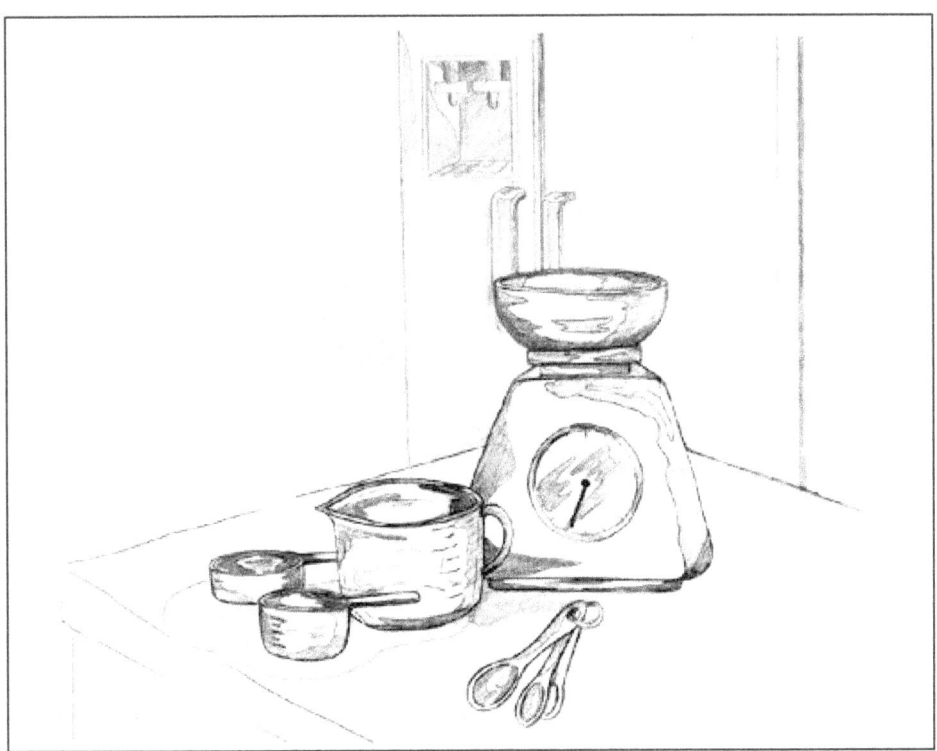

Be careful to keep track of your fluids and other foods.

What do I need to know about potassium?

Potassium is a mineral found in many foods, especially milk, fruits, and vegetables. It affects how steadily your heart beats. Healthy kidneys keep the right amount of potassium in the blood to keep the heart beating at a steady pace. Potassium levels can rise between dialysis sessions and affect your heartbeat. Eating too much potassium can be very dangerous to your heart. It may even cause death.

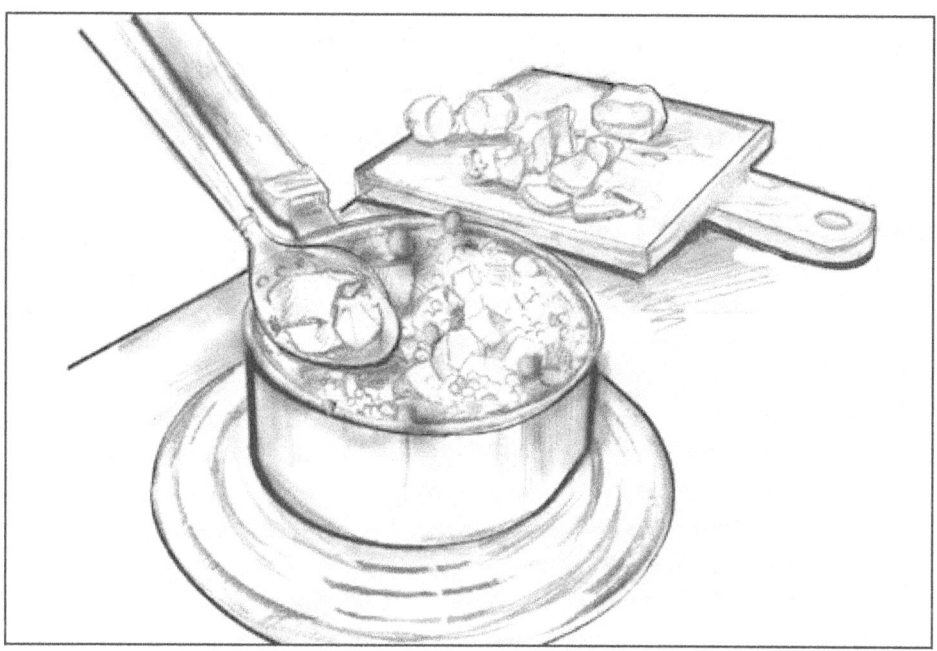

You can remove some potassium from potatoes by dicing or shredding them and then boiling them in water.

To control potassium levels in your blood, avoid foods like avocados, bananas, kiwis, and dried fruit, which are very high in potassium. Also, eat smaller portions of other high-potassium foods. For example, eat half a pear instead of a whole pear. Eat only very small portions of oranges and melons.

Dicing and Boiling Potatoes to Reduce Potassium

You can remove some of the potassium from potatoes by dicing or shredding them and then boiling them in water. Your dietitian will give you more specific information about the potassium content of foods.

Talk With a Dietitian

Make a food plan that reduces the potassium in your diet. Start by noting the high-potassium foods (below) that you now eat. A dietitian can help you add other foods to the list.

High-Potassium Foods:

apricots	kiwi fruit	potatoes
avocados	lima beans	prune juice
bananas	melons	prunes
beets	milk	raisins
Brussels sprouts	nectarines	sardines
cantaloupe	orange juice	spinach
clams	oranges	tomatoes
dates	peanuts	winter squash
figs	pears (fresh)	yogurt

Others: _____

_____

Changes:

Talk with a dietitian about foods you can eat instead of high-potassium foods.

Instead of _____, I will eat _____.

Instead of _____, I will eat _____.

Instead of _____, I will eat _____.

Instead of _____, I will eat _____.

What do I need to know about phosphorus?

Phosphorus is a mineral found in many foods. If you have too much phosphorus in your blood, it pulls calcium from your bones. Losing calcium will make your bones weak and likely to break. Also, too much phosphorus may make your skin itch. Foods like milk and cheese, dried beans, peas, colas, nuts, and peanut butter are high in phosphorus. Usually, people on dialysis are limited to 1/2 cup of milk per day. The renal dietitian will give you more specific information regarding phosphorus.

You probably will need to take a phosphate binder like Renagel, PhosLo, Tums, or calcium carbonate to control the phosphorus in your blood between dialysis sessions. These medications act like sponges to soak up, or bind, phosphorus while it is in the stomach. Because it is bound, the phosphorus does not get into the blood. Instead, it is passed out of the body in the stool.

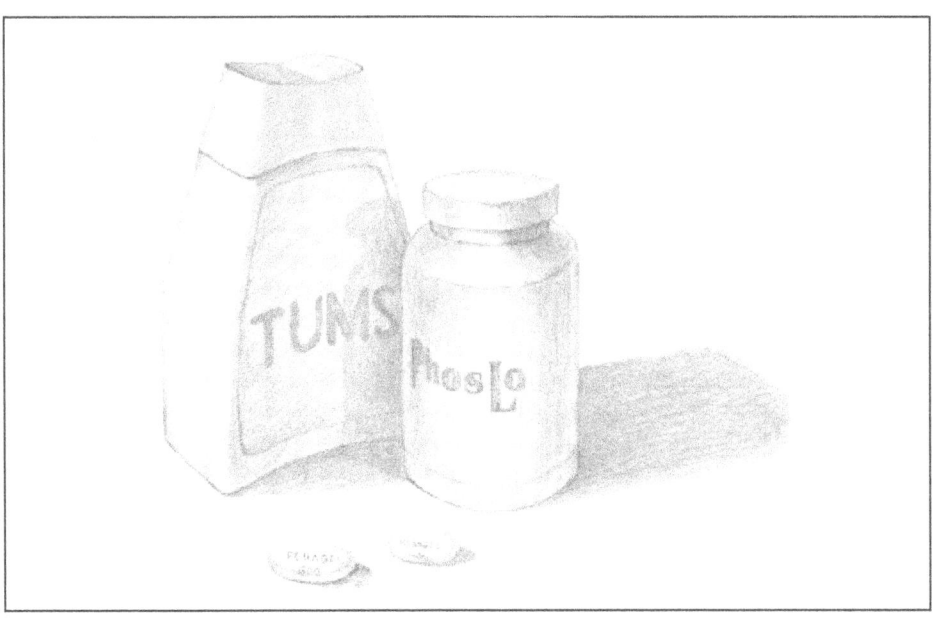

Taking a phosphate binder helps control phosphorus in your blood.

What do I need to know about protein?

Before you were on dialysis, your doctor may have told you to follow a low-protein diet. Being on dialysis changes this. Most people on dialysis are encouraged to eat as much high-quality protein as they can. Protein helps you keep muscle and repair tissue. The better nourished you are, the healthier you will be. You will also have greater resistance to infection and recover from surgery more quickly.

Your body breaks protein down into a waste product called urea. If urea builds up in your blood, it's a sign you have become very sick. Eating mostly high-quality proteins is important because they produce less waste than others. High-quality proteins come from meat, fish, poultry, and eggs (especially egg whites).

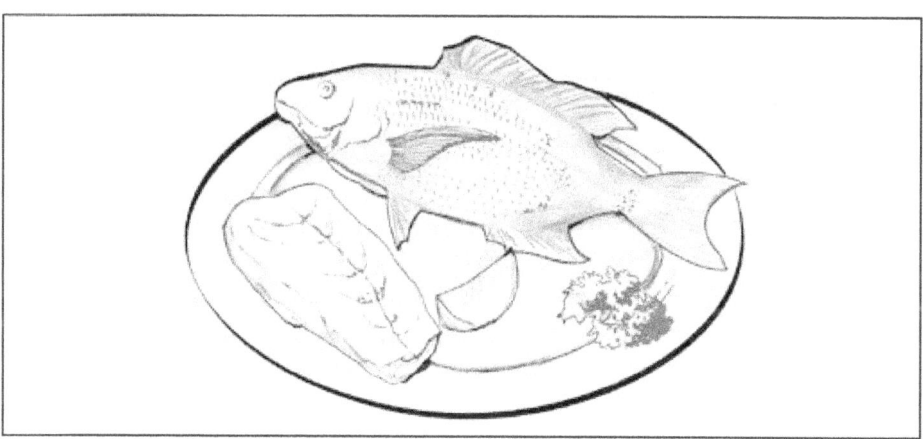

Poultry and fish, like broiled flounder, are good sources of high-quality protein.

Talk With a Dietitian

Meat, fish, and chicken are good sources of protein. Talk with a dietitian about the meats you eat.

I will eat _____ servings of meat each day. A regular serving size is 3 ounces. This is about the size of the palm of your hand or a deck of cards.

Try to choose lean (low-fat) meats that are also low in phosphorus. If you are a vegetarian, ask about other ways to get your protein.

Low-fat milk is a good source of protein. But milk is high in phosphorus and potassium. And milk adds to your fluid intake. Talk with a dietitian to see if milk fits into your food plan.

I (will) (will not) drink milk. I will drink _____ cup(s) of milk a day.

What do I need to know about sodium?

Sodium is found in salt and other foods. Most canned foods and frozen dinners contain large amounts of sodium. Too much sodium makes you thirsty. But if you drink more fluid, your heart has to work harder to pump the fluid through your body. Over time, this can cause high blood pressure and congestive heart failure.

Try to eat fresh foods that are naturally low in sodium. Look for products labeled *low sodium*.

Do not use salt substitutes because they contain potassium. Talk with a dietitian about spices you can use to flavor your food. The dietitian can help you find spice blends without sodium or potassium.

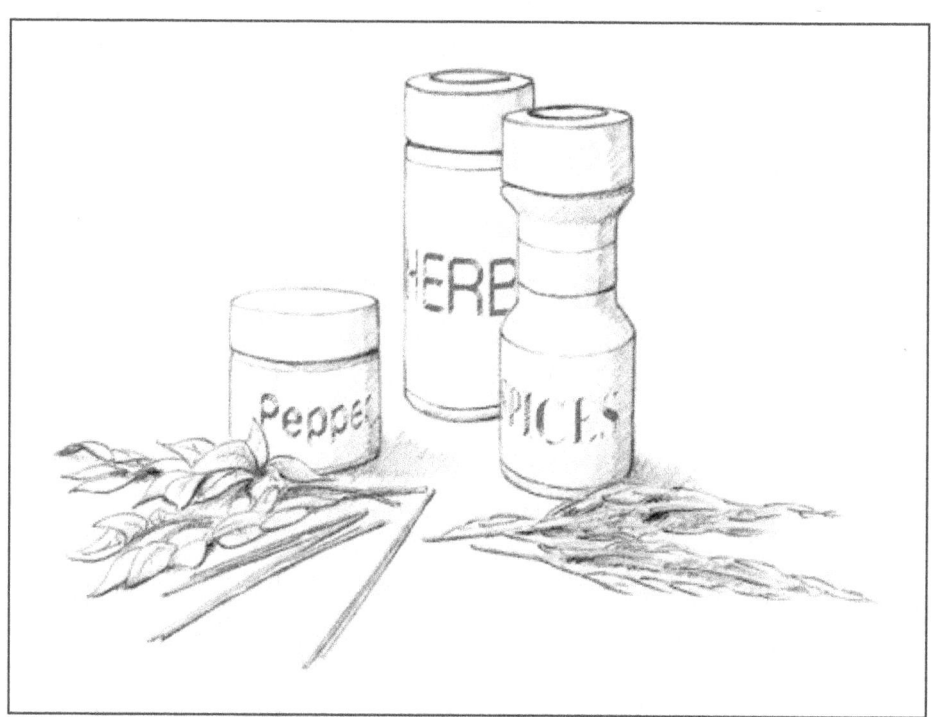

Find new ways to spice up your food.

Talk With a Dietitian

Talk with a dietitian about spices and other healthy foods you can use to flavor your diet. List them on the lines below.

Spice: _____

Spice: _____

Spice: _____

Food: _____

Food: _____

What do I need to know about calories?

Calories provide energy for your body. If your doctor recommends it, you may need to cut down on the calories you eat. A dietitian can help you plan ways to cut calories in the best possible way.

Some people on dialysis need to gain weight. You may need to find ways to add calories to your diet. Vegetable oils—like olive oil, canola oil, and safflower oil—are good sources of calories. Use them generously on breads, rice, and noodles.

Butter and margarines are rich in calories. But these fatty foods can also clog your arteries. Use them less often. Soft margarine that comes in a tub is better than stick margarine. Vegetable oils are the healthiest way to add fat to your diet if you need to gain weight.

Hard candy, sugar, honey, jam, and jelly provide calories and energy without clogging arteries or adding other things that your body does not need. **If you have diabetes, be very careful about eating sweets. A dietitian's guidance is very important for people with diabetes.**

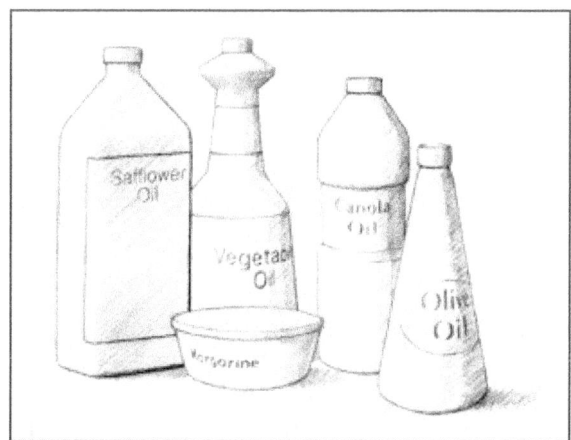

If you need to get extra calories, vegetable oils like these are a good choice.

Should I take vitamins and minerals?

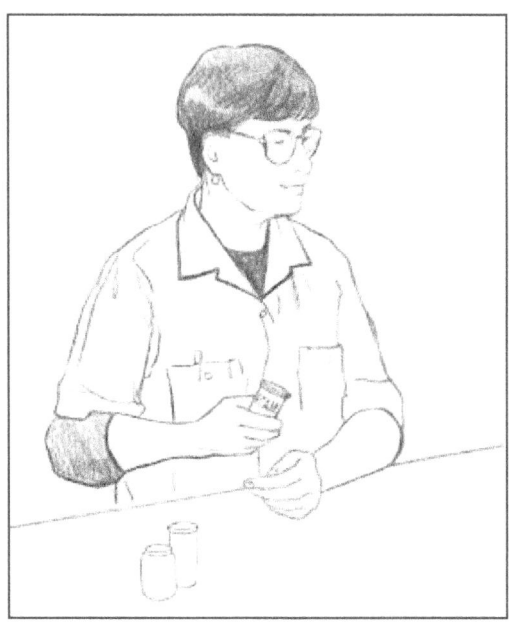

Take only the vitamins your doctor prescribes.

Vitamins and minerals may be missing from your diet because you have to avoid so many foods. Your doctor may prescribe a vitamin and mineral supplement like Nephrocaps.

Warning: Do not take vitamin supplements that you can buy off the store shelf. They may contain vitamins or minerals that are harmful to you.

Resources

Books

Bowes and Church's Food Values of Portions Commonly Used
Eighteenth Edition
Jean A.T. Pennington and Judith S. Douglass
J.P. Lippincott Co. 2004
ISBN: 0–7817–4429–6

The Complete Book of Food Counts
Seventh Edition
Corinne T. Netzer
Dell Publishing Co. 2005
ISBN: 0–440–24123–5

Brochures

Nutrition and Hemodialysis
National Kidney Foundation
30 East 33rd Street
New York, NY 10016
Phone: 1–800–622–9010 or 212–889–2210

How to Increase Calories in Your Renal Diet
National Kidney Foundation
30 East 33rd Street
New York, NY 10016
Phone: 1–800–622–9010 or 212–889–2210

Charts and Posters

Kidney HELPER Phosphorus Guide (chart or poster)
Kidney HELPER Potassium Guide (chart or poster)
Available from Consumer MedHelp, Inc.
2437 Bay Area Boulevard
PMB 128
Houston, TX 77058
Phone: 877–248–2331 or 281–486–9258
Fax: 281–576–8990
Email: info@consumermedhelp.com
Internet: www.consumermedhelp.com

Picture Renal Diet (poster)
Available from University Hospital, Food and Nutrition Services
619 South 19th Street
Birmingham, AL 35233
Phone: 205–934–6375
Internet: www.health.uab.edu

Cookbooks

These cookbooks provide recipes for people on dialysis:

The Renal Gourmet
Mardy Peters
ISBN: 0–9641730–0–X
Emenar Incorporated
13N625 Coombs Road
Elgin, IL 60123
Fax: 847–741–8696
Email: webmaster@kidney-cookbook.com
Internet: www.kidney-cookbook.com

Southwest Cookbook for People on Dialysis
Developed by the El Paso Chapter Council on Renal Nutrition
   and the National Kidney Foundation of Texas, Inc.
Published by a grant from Amgen Inc.
Internet: www.epogen.com/patient/recipes/join_recipeclub-ssl.
   html

Creative Cooking for Renal Diets
Cleveland Clinic Foundation
ISBN: 0–941511–00–6
Senay Publishing
Email: jsenay@adelphia.net
Internet: www.patientsupport.net

Creative Cooking for Renal Diabetic Diets
Cleveland Clinic Foundation
ISBN: 0–941511–01–4
Senay Publishing
P.O. Box 397
Chesterland, OH 44026
Phone: 866–648–2693
Email: jsenay@adelphia.net
Internet: www.patientsupport.net

Cooking for David
Culinary Kidney Cooks
P.O. Box 468
Huntington Beach, CA 92648
Phone: 714–842–4684
Email: Eric.Brooks@CulinaryKidneyCooks.com
Internet: www.culinarykidneycooks.com

More Online Information

The American Association of Kidney Patients provides an online nutrition counter at *www.aakp.org/brochures/nutrition-counter*.

The National Kidney Foundation offers many fact sheets for patients with kidney disease at *www.kidney.org* on the Internet.

Acknowledgments

The individuals listed here provided editorial guidance or facilitated field testing for this publication. The National Kidney and Urologic Diseases Information Clearinghouse would like to thank them for their contribution.

Lawrence Y. Agodoa, M.D.
End-Stage Renal Disease Program
National Institute of Diabetes and Digestive and Kidney Diseases
National Institutes of Health
Bethesda, MD

Kim Bayer, M.A., R.D., L.D.
BMA Dialysis
Bethesda, MD

Josephine P. Briggs, M.D.
Howard Hughes Medical Institute
Chevy Chase, MD

Shirley Cox, R.D., L.D.
Amarillo High Plains Dialysis Center
Amarillo, TX

Sana Dicey, R.D.
Department of Chronic Dialysis Programs
Shore Memorial Hospital
Somers Point, NJ

Laura Byham Gray, M.S., R.D., C.N.S.D.
Department of Nutrition Services
Shore Memorial Hospital
Somers Point, NJ

Linda Hager, M.S., R.D.
Total Renal Care
Minneapolis Dialysis Unit
Minneapolis, MN

Melissa Hildebrand, R.D., L.D.
Total Renal Care
Minneapolis Dialysis Unit
Minneapolis, MN

Lisa Hill, R.D., C.D.E.
Dialysis Clinic, Inc.
Nashville, TN

Jean King, R.D., C.D.E.
Pikes Peak Dialysis Center, Inc.
Colorado Springs, CO

Wanda Knopik
Total Renal Care
Minneapolis Dialysis Unit
Minneapolis, MN

Susan Lindsey-Goldman, R.D.
Kessler Dialysis
Hammonton, NJ

Betty Murray, R.N.
Dialysis Clinic, Inc.
Nashville, TN

Andrew Narva, M.D.
National Kidney Disease Education Program
National Institute of Diabetes and Digestive and Kidney Diseases
National Institutes of Health
Bethesda, MD

Jean Pennington, Ph.D., R.D.
Division of Nutrition Research Coordination
National Institute of Diabetes and Digestive and Kidney Diseases
National Institutes of Health
Bethesda, MD

Gail Radosevich, R.D., L.D.
Total Renal Care
Minneapolis Dialysis Unit
Minneapolis, MN

Susan Schommer, R.D., L.D.
Total Renal Care
Minneapolis Dialysis Unit
Minneapolis, MN

Charlotte Stall, M.A., R.D.
The Children's Hospital
Denver, CO

About the Kidney Failure Series

You and your doctor will work together to choose a treatment that's best for you. The publications of the National Institute of Diabetes and Digestive and Kidney Diseases (NIDDK) Kidney Failure Series can help you learn about the specific issues you will face.

Booklets
- *Eat Right to Feel Right on Hemodialysis*
- *Kidney Failure: Choosing a Treatment That's Right for You*
- *Kidney Failure Glossary*
- *Treatment Methods for Kidney Failure: Hemodialysis*
- *Treatment Methods for Kidney Failure: Peritoneal Dialysis*
- *Treatment Methods for Kidney Failure: Transplantation*

Fact Sheets
- *Amyloidosis and Kidney Disease*
- *Anemia in Kidney Disease and Dialysis*
- *Financial Help for Treatment of Kidney Failure*
- *Hemodialysis Dose and Adequacy*
- *Home Hemodialysis*
- *Kidney Failure: What to Expect*
- *Peritoneal Dialysis Dose and Adequacy*
- *Renal Osteodystrophy*
- *Vascular Access for Hemodialysis*

Learning as much as you can about your treatment will help make you an important member of your health care team.

The NIDDK will develop additional materials for this series as needed. Please address any comments about this series and requests for copies to the National Kidney and Urologic Diseases Information Clearinghouse. Descriptions of the publications in this series are available on the Internet at *www.kidney.niddk.nih.gov/kudiseases/pubs/kidneyfailure/ index.htm.*

National Kidney and Urologic Diseases Information Clearinghouse

3 Information Way
Bethesda, MD 20892–3580
Phone: 1–800–891–5390
TTY: 1–866–569–1162
Fax: 703–738–4929
Email: nkudic@info.niddk.nih.gov
Internet: www.kidney.niddk.nih.gov

The National Kidney and Urologic Diseases Information Clearinghouse (NKUDIC) is a service of the National Institute of Diabetes and Digestive and Kidney Diseases (NIDDK). The NIDDK is part of the National Institutes of Health of the U.S. Department of Health and Human Services. Established in 1987, the Clearinghouse provides information about diseases of the kidneys and urologic system to people with kidney and urologic disorders and to their families, health care professionals, and the public. The NKUDIC answers inquiries, develops and distributes publications, and works closely with professional and patient organizations and Government agencies to coordinate resources about kidney and urologic diseases.

Publications produced by the Clearinghouse are carefully reviewed by both NIDDK scientists and outside experts.

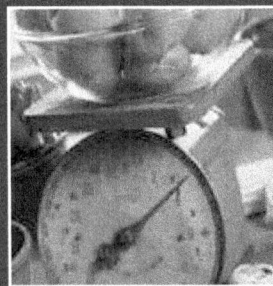

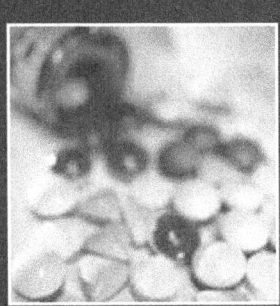

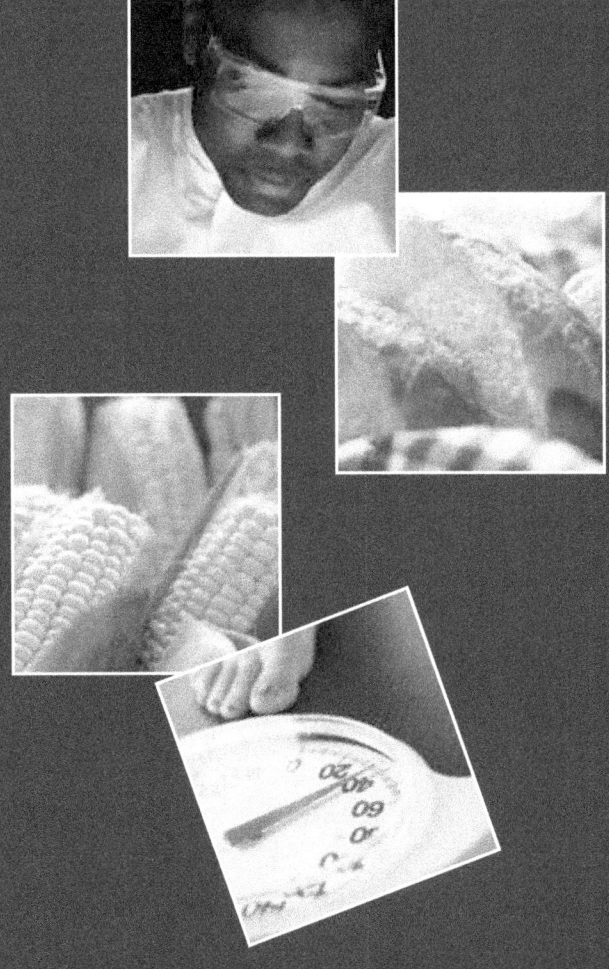

 U.S. Department of Health and Human Services
National Institutes of Health

NIDDK | NATIONAL INSTITUTE OF
DIABETES AND DIGESTIVE
AND KIDNEY DISEASES

NIH Publication No. 08–4274

August 2008